Mom Just Wants to Go Home

WISHES, REALITY, AND RESOURCES

LYNDA JAMES-GILBOE

ISBN 978-1-66789-868-1

eBook ISBN 978-1-66789-869-8

Dedicated to…

My family

John, for always having my back no matter what

Kevin, Emily, Morgan, and Laura, Alexandra, and Sloane, I love you

Mom and Dad, I did my best

TABLE OF CONTENTS

FORWARD

You may have heard about the Medicare "donut hole," the limbo you're in during some years when your own spending and your plan's spending reaches a predetermined amount. You don't leave the donut hole until your spending reaches the catastrophic coverage level. While this has created big financial hardships for many families over the years, there is another gap in the healthcare system that feels more like the Grand Canyon than a donut hole.

Elderly people who need some type of assistance to either stay in their own home or to move to assisted living facilities can face real financial challenges since these services are not typically covered by Medicare/Medicaid. Depending on where you live, there are some waiver programs that can help a bit, but you may encounter long waiting lists. When such individuals require nursing home care, Medicaid may come to the rescue and pay for nursing home care. But when you face a situation in which your loved one really needs more help but doesn't need a nursing home or strongly prefers to remain at home, you enter the haves/have not zone.

There are some wonderful, assisted living options out there, but costs are high for basic rent and additional health care options offered on site may be priced ala carte. In looking into options for my own Mom,

I encountered pricing from $12-75K plus just for rent annually, with the low range being a group home -type setting. Similarly, at-home care is very expensive, and can run anywhere between $15-$30 per hour. I firmly believe these home care workers deserve this pay and more; it's just not affordable to many Americans to pay this kind of money. To have someone in the home just four hours a day is more than $20,000 per year minimum, and for many, four hours, or even one person, is not enough. I'd like to pause here and express my thanks and appreciation to A Place for Mom, a truly wonderful organization who works hard to help people find a good solution for their loved ones. When I reached out to them, the person who assisted me was thoughtful and caring, and I'm grateful. And I was pleased to learn that they are able to help with options for either at-home care or finding a new place for loved ones to live. But even this terrific service can only go so far for seniors with limited financial resources.

When she joined Medicare, my mom took care to pick a good Medigap plan, but ultimately that didn't cover many of the services she came to need. And her savings would not cover even a partial year of assisted living or at-home care service. My siblings and I are retired or approaching retirement ourselves and prices for these services would quickly dilute or even wipe out our own retirement savings, particularly scary given the uncertainty one hears about the future of the Social Security system. Draining our savings and perpetrating this problem for our own children does not seem like a good answer.

So, what does this mean? People like my mom, and I bet there are a lot of them in the United States, do the best they can to live their lives, relying on family and friends to help keep it all together. But as infirmities progress, this gets harder and harder to maintain. The notion of relying on elderly adult children to assist their even more elderly parents with daily living tasks like showering, getting up and down, and the hundreds of things we all need to do every day is physically and emotionally daunting, and can become overwhelming, or simply impossible to maintain. Relationships can become permanently strained. In other cases, there really isn't anyone available who can offer this kind of help, so the elderly person is fending for themselves.

The bottom line is this. You're fine if you don't have any need for home care or assisted living. You're also likely fine, or at least more financially stable, if you do need nursing home care as you can apply for Medicaid if you don't have financial resources or long-term care insurance to pay for it. **But if you need home care or assisted living, and don't have a way to fund those things privately, you will quickly find yourself at the bottom of the Grand Canyon, with no way up.**

The toll of navigating through this enormous chasm of minimal and non-assistance is tremendous. The stress of worrying about loved ones who need more help but can't get it is massive. The risk of injury or emotional impact related to living in this gap is always there and growing and impacts both the elderly family member and the care givers.

This story is about my own family's experience of living in this gap for years. I have not tried to provide formal research statistics or data about trends, this is a personal story. But I do know this – we are not unique in this journey. Too many seniors face poverty, live in fear, and aren't getting the help they need. And their families face stress and worry as they try to help.

In my own parents' case, I will be the first to admit that they have some culpability for the situation in which they found themselves in their later years. I'll talk about that in the Prologue. At the same time, even if they had made better choices at several junctures, it is unlikely they could have covered all of the expenses for the care that they ultimately needed. I can vouch for the fact that the possibility of outliving resources is a real and scary phenomenon, adding complexity and fear to the final days of some people. And navigating through the services that do exist can be mind-boggling. Even Medicare with all that it offers requires some real study and analysis to get the best plan. Sorting through the plans can be mind-numbing and really hard to understand for even the most experienced and plugged-in seniors.

Before I begin, I'd like to share an internal struggle I faced as I wrote this. Some of this content is raw and painful. I know my parents would be unhappy with me for telling this story – they had a very firm rule about "dirty laundry" always staying within the family. I'm sorry to break this rule, but I concluded that the truth about this very difficult time in our lives doesn't diminish the good things they did or their lifelong value. Sugar-coating helps no one. These issues are real, not shameful. Many families face these challenges, and too much of what I read about this long-term care assistance gap speaks glowingly about how heroic family members bridge this gap with financial and personal sacrifice and the "privilege" of helping elderly parents, without seriously contemplating systemic changes that are urgently needed. That's the shameful part – that families are at risk, facing exhaustion, and financial difficulties as they try to help their elderly members. The healthcare system is broken and support options for the aging are just another example of that.

PROLOGUE

My parents got married in the fifties right out of high school and were together more than sixty years. They raised four kids and had a good life together. My dad was very smart, with a strong entrepreneurial spirit. He was a dreamer. He wanted to be in business for himself and started several businesses while I was growing up…a fuel oil distribution business, an A&W drive-in, a combination party store/fast-food chicken store, and a discount pop/beer store. He loved coming up with the ideas and getting things set up and my very artistic mom worked with him in these undertakings. She did all sorts of things to help, but her specialty was creating signage. Ultimately, though, he was less interested in the day-to-day running of these businesses, and each ended over time.

He never really made "the killing" that he hoped to make and was open about having no retirement plans. He used to say, "I'll never live beyond 65 anyway." Planning to die is, of course, not a plan, and even as a worrywart kid, it made me uneasy about the future to hear him say this, especially since I witnessed the health challenges my own grandparents had faced.

In the latter part of his working life, he took a series of jobs that covered expenses and that even allowed my parents to save a little. Dad was an avid reader of the *Wall Street Journal* and was very interested in the stock market. They moved to Florida, and my younger sister bought a house right next door to them. One day while visiting all of them, my sister and our families went to one of the Florida amusement parks. My sister turned to me while we were waiting in line for a ride, and whispered, "Mom told me that Dad lost all of their savings on a bad stock purchase." He had once again been in search of making "a killing," and had bet the farm and lost it all with no way to make it up.

We all carried on and no one really talked about it and just kept our fingers crossed. My sister kept an eye on things and even helped dad find a job that he enjoyed in his late sixties. But that came to an end when he had his first stroke. Social Security and Medicare kept the wheels on the bus for a while. When my sister and brother-in-law found that their family was expanding from two kids to four kids since twins were on the way, they decided to build a new house a block over from my parents. And thinking ahead, they generously included a first-floor bathroom and den that could be converted for my parents should the day arrive in which staying in their own home wouldn't be an option.

Then tragedy struck. My sister gave birth to the twins and died the same day. She was only 37 and her loss is felt to this day. My parents were never the same. Wanting someone to blame, they lashed out at those around them and decided to move from Florida back to their home state of Michigan. Their vision of growing old with my younger sister nearby was blown forever. They were stuck with me, the workaholic daughter, and their two sons, to help them navigate the future. They asked me to find them an apartment and gave me specific criteria about what they wanted in terms of features and pricing. I fulfilled their requests precisely, and at the time, they were still managing their expenses, and so I had no real insight into the amount of money they received from Social Security or their specific monthly expenses. They did get some money from the sale of their house.

I also didn't know that my mom had begun seeing more and more signs that my dad wasn't tracking well. He'd always been a bit opinionated and prone to controversial thinking, so we kids didn't notice the changes to the same extent as my mom did. Prices at the apartment kept rising as did other expenses, and over the next eight years, my husband and I began taking on more and more of their monthly expenses. Even then, though, we didn't have the benefit of the full picture or how much they had left, but we tried hard to help. It's now clear that my mom knew that things were not good, but my dad didn't accept that and didn't want to discuss it. As it turns out, we learned that his strokes were contributing to vascular dementia, which continued to worsen over time. For his part, I think his plan continued to be to die before his money ran out.

Things came to a head when they were notified that the Medigap Part C prices increased substantially. My parents placed a high value on having "good" insurance, as do I, and really wanted to keep their plan just the way it was. My mom showed me the letter because she was worried, and while I didn't have their total financial picture, intuitively I thought this was alarming. I pressed them for more details. My dad insisted that they could handle this, and also insisted that I was not understanding the new price, claiming that it would be much less. When I finally got the full picture and confirmed the pricing structure, I realized that not only could they not absorb this increase, that they had very little of their savings left from the sale of their home. It also became clear to me that my dad was not thinking rationally. My mom hadn't wanted to upset him and let him remain as the main financial decision maker for too long. Further, my husband and I had been increasingly concerned about the amount of money we were contributing to their household expenses each month as we contemplated our own looming retirement. We had made solid retirement plans, but they didn't include supporting my parents to this extent.

In an effort to get my parents' expenses under control while also stopping the bleeding for us, my husband and I decided to use a portion of our retirement savings to buy a house for them to live in. This would allow them to live without a rent payment and within their Social Security monthly payments. And our own expenses would be contained as well to taxes and insurance, or so we thought. And then some day in the distant future, the idea was that we would sell the house and return the money to our own retirement savings. That was the plan we embarked on.

We found a small house and worked on getting it set up. We converted the bathroom so that it would be accessible and added new appliances and ramps outside. Although we were not going to charge them rent, we found ourselves subject to all sorts of rules and regulations as "landlords" from the city and insurance companies which made an already difficult project even harder. But we got it done. Then a week before their scheduled move-in, my dad fell and broke his hip.

Sadly, he never really recovered. He had surgery and was sent to rehab, but his disorientation and dementia quickly accelerated. Because it was abundantly clear that he needed nursing home care, we were able to successfully apply for Medicaid on his behalf, and most expenses were taken care of. While I didn't realize it then, the experience with my dad provided a window into the future with my mom. She asked me to take care of all of the arrangements, the paperwork, and even told the facility to call me whenever there were decisions to make about my dad's care. It was a sad time, but at least we had a plan and a way to deal with the financial aspect. However, there was another financial hit waiting for my mom when he died five months later. Her household Social Security income was now less. She had a twenty-year old car and all sorts of medical issues of her own, including diabetes. She'd had one knee replaced, but not gotten around to doing the other, so had serious mobility challenges. She moved into the house by herself, and we added a medical alert service to help ensure she could get help should she need it.

I'm pleased and grateful to say that things went along pretty well for an additional five years. Mom settled in and family members all worked together to ensure that she had groceries, prescriptions, and some light housekeeping help. I did try to get her plugged into some services that the local senior community center offered like rides to appointments, but she wasn't interested, she wanted family to help her. We had regular family get-togethers at her house, to make it easier for her to stay connected to everyone, and even hosted a couple of Zoom calls from her house during the pandemic! She had a few mishaps during those years in which she called emergency services, including the time she was trying to open a pickle jar and pressed the jar against the call-button pendant she wears around her neck, but all-in-all, she managed reasonably well.

But then things began to change. The health scares increased. We began seeing that she wasn't tracking her bills as carefully. Sometimes she was unsure if she took her medicine. She was eating poorly. Her family became concerned about various aspects of daily living like daily hygiene and shower safety. And to make matters even more complicated, she vehemently denied there were any issues, insisting that everything was fine as it was.

And this is where this story begins. In November 2021, my family and I ran headlong into the massive gap in the availability of services to elderly who have limited financial resources, and who prefer to stay in their home. We also encountered endless rules. Some of these rules were privacy-related and intended to protect my mom's rights. As more than one person said to us, "as long as she is alert and oriented, she has the right to make her own decisions, even if they are bad ones." And unfortunately, even as we tried to help her, she battled us every step of the way, insisting that there was nothing to be concerned about. We did our best to navigate this chasm, but the stress inflicted has been immeasurable for my mom, for me, and for our entire family.

CHAPTER 1

FIRST SIGNS OF TROUBLE

One morning in early November 2021, my husband and I were awakened in our Florida home by an emergency call. My mother in Michigan had fallen, she was disoriented, and was initially unable to provide her address or the names of her children to the emergency responders who had been called by her medical alert service. My brother met the paramedics, and we all talked on the phone. The paramedics described an alarming scene, pills spilled all over the living room floor, and food spilled in the kitchen. My mother was resisting being taken to the hospital. My brother and I agreed with the paramedics that she needed to go.

My brother went with her to the hospital, and I got a plane from Florida to Michigan, scheduled to arrive later that same day. COVID was still making things challenging at hospitals at the time and my brother could not go in with her. He was told to check back in a couple of hours. When he returned, he learned that she had an infection, would be prescribed an antibiotic, and was expected to leave immediately! With great trepidation, given her condition just hours earlier, he took her back home, and got her settled back in the house.

When I landed, I picked up something for her for dinner, picked up her new prescription, and made sure she took her meds. I made an appointment with her regular doctor to follow-up. While scheduling the appointment, I emphasized that we had concerns about her living alone. The appointment was scheduled for four days away.

Within a couple of days, she was struggling with side-effects of the antibiotic, and refused to continue taking it. So, she had a new malady, and was using nothing to fight the original severe infection until we saw the doctor. Given my mom's mobility issues, when it came time to take her to the doctor, I had difficulty getting her into the car. She was unable to lift her feet on her own. At the doctor's office, it was apparent that she wouldn't be able to make it back to the exam room, even using her walker, so they used a wheelchair. Her doctor did a good job of asking her some probing questions about life at home and how things like showering, meal preparation, and so on were going. Unfortunately, she said everything was fine, and would not admit there were any issues. I tried to respectfully provide clarifying information at a couple of points. For example, I knew that she was experiencing some intimate physical problems, but she insisted there were no issues when the doctor asked.

This question of how best to navigate the important need to honor privacy and maintain dignity while actually addressing very real health and intimate health concerns became an ongoing area of concern as time went on. And my mother was an especially difficult case, since she just wouldn't engage at all about certain things or would provide answers that were not truthful.

Fortunately, during that visit, the doctor prescribed another antibiotic to mitigate the side-effects of her first antibiotic and did a good job of reading between the lines. She prescribed some home nursing checks and physical therapy. I was so relieved! My mom was so exhausted at the end of the visit that I called my brother to help me get her back into the house.

I had no doubt that it would be completely impossible for me to hold her up if she started to fall, and I didn't want to risk that.

While I was glad that the doctor had prescribed help, I was a little concerned about whether this would stick since my mother had not gotten along well with a previous home care agency we tried, saying she didn't like people in the house and that they were stealing from her. (There was no evidence of that.) After another few days, I returned to Florida, expecting that she would at least give the extra help a try, as she said she would. Unfortunately, not only did it not stick, but it never even started because when they called her to set up appointments, she told them not to come.

Things bumped along uneasily for another few months. More of her bills were not paid on time. When I talked to her about it, she blamed the post office. And in fairness to her, I suspect there is some truth in that, as first-class mail does take a while to arrive these days. But it was happening too often. She incurred a late charge on her credit card. I was especially worried about her medigap supplement payments. I worked on getting most of her bills on autopay to help eliminate this worry.

When she stopped working with the senior agency who supplied housekeeping assistance for a couple of hours each week, my daughter took this on, and cleaned her house every Sunday, as she refused to consider any non-family options. My daughter began finding extremely soiled towels, bedding, and even floor areas. I sent regular Amazon shipments to make sure that there would be extras of these things so that she could just discard heavily soiled items if they were too much to deal with. (I was so proud of my daughter as she did this difficult work. She told me once that "I remind myself that grandma changed me when I was little, and I just jump in and try not to think about what I'm actually doing.") Garbage was thrown in the sink or in bags hanging from her walker, including soiled incontinence pads. Once a week help didn't seem enough, but we had no other good options. My daughter is a single-mom who works full time, and one-day a week was all she could manage. Even if Mom would agree to it, home care is very expensive, and her resources continued to dwindle.

Mom has always been an avid Kindle reader and used it to make Amazon purchases. I was always pleased that she could do this so easily until I discovered that she had spent almost $400 in one month on non-essential items. When I say "non-essential," I'm really just talking about in the context of need and budget. If I had my druthers, I would want my mom to be able to purchase anything that made her happy, as long as it wasn't dangerous or harmful. Unfortunately, among other things, she was spending a lot of money on snacks that were not healthy for someone with diabetes. So not only was she was damaging her financial viability, but she was also literally impacting her physical wellbeing with these purchases.

My daughter and I devised a system for getting her groceries. Mom would write out her list, my daughter would enter her order through an online grocery delivery service, and then I would work to answer any questions the shopper had about the order, including replacement questions. With increasing frequency, Mom would include items that she already had in the house, and when that happened, my daughter just edited them out of the order. The shopper would deliver the groceries to a chair just inside the front door and my mom would then take the better part of the week to put them away. She focused on things that needed to go in the freezer and refrigerator first. Unfortunately, we began to find things in the refrigerator that should go in the freezer. It was necessary to do periodic purges to get rid of items that had expired or hadn't been stored properly.

I had always visited Michigan frequently, but began visiting even more often, well outside what my budget had been built to sustain. Each time, I arrived feeling uneasy and left feeling the same way or more worried. My mother continued to deny there were any issues and rebuffed even simple things that might help her. When I noticed that she had trouble taking care of her toenails, I got her a foot massager to soften them and special clippers for seniors. She wouldn't soak her feet, even when I offered to set it up for her while I was there. When my brother took her to a podiatrist in an effort to take care of her nails, she did it once, but told him there is no way she would go back.

CHAPTER 2

THE POT ROAST SAGA

Mom had a system for working in the kitchen. She had become mostly a microwave user and would sit on the seat of her walker to move between the refrigerator, the microwave, and the sink. She kept many groceries out on the table for easy access. One day in March 2022, she was trying to get something out of the freezer that she wanted to microwave. In the process of pulling out the item she wanted, a heavy frozen pot roast became dislodged and flew out of the freezer and hit the top of her foot hard.

The foot did not seem to be broken, but it was very bruised and quickly became discolored. It was painful and compromised her mobility even further. During that same period, I had already been reminding her to get a doctor's appointment since her prescriptions were coming up for refill. Her pattern had been to resist going to the doctor unless essential, and thank goodness, she considered prescriptions essential, and she knew they wouldn't be refilled without a visit. My intuition is that she really didn't want to go this time because she would have to tell the doctor that she ignored the home help that she had prescribed in her previous visit. (She once had a doctor "fire" her as a patient for ignoring her care plan.) Her doctor is actually a very relaxed easy-going woman, but she likely would have at least asked her about her progress since her last visit, and Mom probably wasn't keen to have that discussion.

All her kids and grandkids urged her to get the appointment as soon as possible, both to get her prescriptions renewed and to have the doctor take a look at her foot. While I was back in Florida, I did the same, noting that it could be pretty dangerous for her should the foot get infected. It was my understanding that feet are especially vulnerable for diabetics, and I didn't want her to risk losing the foot.

Finally, one afternoon, she called me and asked me to give her the phone number of her doctor, as she couldn't find it. She said her foot was looking worse and she thought there was an infection that might be going up to her ankle. I was horrified and quickly got her the number. She did call for an appointment and my brother took her. The doctor took one look at the foot and said that she needed to be hospitalized immediately as an IV of antibiotics was essential to fight the infection. She told me later that her heart sank when she heard that, as she figured that she would just get a prescription and be on her way.

She was admitted to the hospital where she remained for several days to get the infection under control. After four days, the foot was looking better, but she had lost strength overall, and was considered a fall risk. She could not get out of bed or walk without help.

I had flown up from Florida and was in her hospital room when the discharge coordinator stopped by her room to plan her discharge. The hospital said she needed to go to a rehab facility to get her strength back before she could safely go home. On the care coordinator's advice, we looked at Medicare.gov to find some nearby facility options, with the criteria being to pick someplace that had a high number of "stars." And we also wanted to avoid the one where my dad had died, given the sadness of that time. I found two five-star facilities and we picked the one nearest my mom's house. I reminded Mom that this place had been our first choice for dad when he needed care, but there had been no availability at the time. It would also be convenient for family members to visit. I went to see it, and it looked very nice. She was then scheduled to be transported over, and that's when the nightmare really began.

CHAPTER 3

YOU'RE TAKING AWAY MY RIGHTS!

lthough all of us could see that mom could not even get out of bed without help, and the hospital had flagged her as a fall risk, she refused to accept that she needed rehab work. The morning following her admission, she called me early and demanded that I come and get her and take her home. She told me that I owed it to her given all the things she had done for me during my life. When I tried to reason with her, she hung up on me. The reality is that I could not have taken her home even if I wanted to. She could not walk; I could not lift her. Leaving her alone in her home in her current state was not even remotely an option, in my mind. And of course, the whole point of rehab was to get her strength back so she could safely go home.

Over the next couple of weeks, she alternated between doing the rehab work she needed, while also periodically calling me and demanding I take her back to her house. Her treatment of me became increasingly abusive, especially on the phone, although that moved to in-person as time went on. I was in town for much of April and visited her every day when I was there. She somehow concluded that because her injury wasn't caused by a fall, she didn't need the therapy, never accepting the point that she was weakened by her inactivity at home and in the hospital. She told us that she really could get around and that the only reason she didn't is that the facility wouldn't let her, and she was being held back. It is certainly true that the facility had flagged her difficulties in getting up and down and required that she have help. Her mobility issues were evident every time I visited. She struggled with dressing. Even things like moving her legs back into bed after sitting on the side could not be done without help. Yet, she blamed me for her being in rehab, saying that she was being kept there for my convenience. She evidently needed a punching bag, and I was elected. While this was all incredibly difficult for her, I can say definitively that "convenient" is not a word that describes this experience for me.

During this period, she said horrible things to me directly and about me to others that I will never be able to forget. Words really do take a toll. At the time, I was still working, and juggling those responsibilities while having my mother call me and tell me that if I didn't take her home that day, her wish for me was that I would die in a nursing home, and then have to pop back into a conference call, was devastatingly hard. She told my daughter that she wanted to punch me when she visited her on Easter and brought her some flowers from me. I began to realize that it was possible that my mom could die someday feeling only hatred for me. I told myself that if I have to choose between my mom being happy with me or being safe, I have to choose safe. But the situation was profoundly sad. Why was this on me? Why wouldn't she talk about the situation, consider options, and accept that she had some responsibility here? The stress was palpable. And after a few weeks, it was clear that proceeding with my plans to scale back my work was the best course of action for several reasons but managing the unpredictability of the issues with my mom was a real factor.

This might be a moment to digress. My parents were from a different time and neither of them ever showed much interest in my career or understood why it was important to me. I was an A student in high school and earned college scholarships, including one four-year full ride option. When I was in my teens, my dad spoke about my college plans in the context of going to "get my MRS degree." (As it turned out, I married a man I met in high school and never used "Mrs." as part of my name.) As my career progressed, I traveled extensively and loved it. They never liked this, saying it was unsafe, and asking why this was necessary. While this story is not about me, there is an irony here. My crazy job was actually the reason I was able to provide the help they came to need, but I don't think they ever really saw that. I believe they loved all of their children, including me, but family discussions about feelings or emotions were always off the table. Mom wanted to stay in "tell mode" and order me to take her home, rather than to discuss options and plan together. She consistently rebuffed all efforts to do that.

During this period Mom spoke with an 83-year-old extended family member, with whom she was close, each night on the phone. To ensure confidentiality, and for simplicity's sake, I'll call this person "Louise." Given the pandemic, Louise had not actually seen Mom in well over a year and did not know the full details of her extensive list of health issues and did not question my mom's assertions that she was fine, that she could get up and down readily, and that she was managing well. Nor could she witness the daily struggles my mom was having in doing simple things like getting dressed and the episodes of headaches and nausea that caused concern as well. She was not the one running to the nurse's station for crackers and ginger ale when Mom was feeling lightheaded or helping her get dressed or the many other things her kids were doing. She accepted my mom's stance that she did not need rehab and the two of them concluded together that Mom was somehow being held there against her will. I learned that Louise, whom Mom had always said was a bit of a know-it-all, told her that her rights were being violated by her children. This time, though, Mom was listening to her and appeared to have lost the objectivity she'd had in the past about Louise's pronouncements.

This came out about three weeks into her stay. The physical therapist called me to discuss how things were going in advance of a care conference that was, ironically, intended to plan her discharge. Mom's efforts in physical therapy were inconsistent, and the therapist expressed concern that given the state of her progress in physical therapy, coupled with the fact that one knee is bone-on-bone, it is inevitable that she would fall again. She was recommending assisted living or home care. While very concerned about the costs, this made sense to me from a safety perspective, given what we had seen with her progress, especially around doing things like getting up and down. I was fearful about the idea of Mom going home without more help and was very worried about her safety in this next life chapter.

I immediately called A Place for Mom to get some options in advance of the care conference. They were extremely helpful and provided several different paths, including both assisted living and home health care options. Most had affordability issues, but I also learned about a waiver program in Michigan that would potentially cover some of the assistance that my mother might need. I got the ball rolling on looking into the waiver since there is a long waiting list. And it is further complicated by the qualifying criteria of having less than $2000 in assets. Since she still had a bit more than that, we would have to take the plunge without knowing for sure that she would be approved for the waiver when she reached the asset criteria. My thought was that we could use a combination of the little money that she had left, along with additional money that my husband and I would chip in, while we got her settled, and (hopefully) the waiver would kick in. Nerve-wracking, but what choice did we have?

Given my mother's track record of avoiding home care options, I thought it would be good idea to try looking at the assisted living options because that would allow her to maintain her own living space but have the benefit of people who could help around-the-clock should the need arise, so I made some appointments to do so. My mom and I gathered with the care team for the care conference and the team went through the status and expressed their concern about her going home alone without more help, and said they really recommended trying assisted living or at least having home care. I mentioned that I'd made some appointments to look at assisted living options. My mother's reaction was instantaneous; she was furious. She literally bent her head down in the meeting and refused to engage any further. When I made the point that we needed to talk about this, she said "I've lost my rights, you've already made all of the decisions." Of course, no decisions had been made. She turned and began wheeling away in her wheelchair. The rehab center team and I were left sitting there and were unable to have a meaningful discussion, reach any conclusions or finalize plans for her discharge.

Although she refused to discuss anything in the meeting, later that day I did follow-up on the assisted living options, some of which were mind-blowingly expensive. I found that many use an ala carte pricing approach in which you pay rent and also pay for the specific services you need. I thought this was scary because it would be difficult to predict total cash outlay, particularly until/if she was approved for the waiver. Nevertheless, given the circumstances, I was willing to take the financial risk and took a chance on reserving a cute one-bedroom apartment with a balcony. I thought maybe I could convince her to give it a try once we took a look at the floor plans together. That never came to be.

That night, my mom called my brother and demanded he bring her house keys, checkbook, and credit card. Apparently, she'd decided to ignore me completely. After our discharge planning meeting, Mom called Louise who apparently implied that her children may have used up her money. What money? Again, it appears that Louise was overlaying some wild assumptions about my mother's health and financial viability that had no basis in fact. (Actually, the amount of our own money that we have spent to help my mom and dad over the years far exceeds her remaining funds by many multiples.) And the logic of saying we've used up her money, as we are literally contemplating spending even more of our own money will forever escape me. In any event, she said that Louise would be picking her up and taking her home, and she would "get a man" to unlock it if she had to. My brother assured her that her money was where she left it but told her he is not in a position to give her the key to the house as she does not actually own it, and she would need to discuss this with me. She was not happy with this response.

Once we learned of this conversation, my husband called Louise in an effort to talk things through. She said that it is clear that we are not working in my mother's best interests and that we were "illegally attempting to institutionalize her," and hung up. Through their nightly conversations, the two of them had created an alternative view of reality that bore little resemblance to the truth but was fueling increasingly negative thinking and hurtful and self-destructive behavior from my mom.

The following day, my two brothers and I visited Mom again and tried to talk about it, but we couldn't get through. She wasn't interested in talking with us. She told me that since it wasn't her house, she would be getting out, maybe to a hotel or to live with Louise. I tried to talk about how this was just not feasible but was not successful. I did bring her the key she requested. Although she paid no rent, she was a legal tenant, and I thought treating her with that respect was the best course of action, since even if she intended to move, all of her belongings were in the house. I felt withholding the key would have been akin to treating her like a child, and I didn't want to do that, but I still second guess myself and wonder if that would have helped make it harder for her to continue the self-destructive behavior. That said, I also feared that not giving Mom the key would encourage Louise to step up the rhetoric and wanted to try to keep some kind of communication open. Mom said she wanted nothing more to do with any of us and that she would take over working with the center herself on her discharge planning. She told us to leave. When I pressed and asked if she was truly willing to put aside her entire family after 65 years, she said she was.

I can only guess that being angry with me was her way of avoiding the realities of her physical condition and dismissing the advice and help of those around her. By maintaining the stance that she didn't need any help, she didn't accept the help that was available, and sadly, it seems likely that she hindered her own opportunities to improve and stay engaged.

She literally kicked her entire family out of her life, without a backward glance. On our way out, we did update the care coordinator about this unbelievable turn of events. It seemed unfathomable that Mom could be thinking clearly and behave in this way, but again the point was made that when someone is articulate and saying what they want, their direction is followed. So, her discharge planning was now in her hands.

My brothers and I stood in the parking lot of the rehab facility, shell-shocked. One of them said, "I can't believe how quickly she wrote us off." It was a family tragedy of the first order. I had no good ideas about what to do next.

I had originally planned to remain in Michigan for a few more days to make sure all of the discharge plans were in place, whether to assisted living or back home with help, but found an earlier flight and returned home to Florida, with no clue as to how things would unfold.

Thelma and Louise make a plan

It occurred to me that I should reach out to Louise's kids. While I hadn't been in touch with them in decades, I had heard about them from my mom. She told me that Louise was annoyed with her own kids because they were concerned about her driving, and they were always bugging her about going to the doctor. Louise had not been to a doctor in over 50 years and did not believe in the value of doing so. Mom had told me on more than one occasion in the past that "Louise isn't good around sick people." These comments were made as Mom described Louise's reaction to the news that one of their extended group of friends was ill or had died. It seems likely that this aversion to medical care services influenced her thinking about the need for my mom to have medical care.

I'm sure my mom similarly aired her grievances about her own kids. I used to think this this "kid bashing" was harmless and no big deal. I was glad that my mom and Louise were able to talk so often. But now I thought it might be a good idea to share the bigger picture in case their mom was discussing the situation with them. I wanted them to have a broader perspective if possible.

They checked in with their mom and learned that she believed my mom did not need the rehab services and that we, her children, were indeed intent on ensuring that she never go home. No one, including my mom, has ever articulated why they think our stance would suddenly change after all these years. After all, we had purchased the house specifically for my parents to use. But her refusal to interact or discuss things in a meaningful way left us in a difficult spot. They also gave me a heads up that my mom had asked Louise to rent her a one-bedroom apartment, and that she intended to look into it for her. I walked them through why this wouldn't be even remotely financially feasible, not to mention having no one teed up to do all of the things she has been relying on family to do. And who would pack her up? Move her? Set up utilities? She hadn't thought any of it through. And interestingly, neither my mom nor Louise noticed that she had not even considered these items, and certainly had no plan or resources for getting them done. She was shifting a request she might have made to me, to Louise instead.

Then one day, I found a text from one of Louise's daughters saying that her mom had told her that she would be taking my mom home to the house on Friday, May 6. Of course, this is counter to what Mom told me would be her plan was the last time I saw her, that she planned to move to a hotel or in with Louise. (One of her daughters assured me that Louise had no intent to have Mom move in with her, so we are not sure where that was even coming from.) Mom did not let me, or my brothers know about her new plan at all. In addition to our concerns for her own safety, as owners of the house, we were concerned about having her (or anyone) in our property without proper plans to ensure basic safety.

We made the decision to notify Adult Protective Services (APS) if this did, in fact, happen, as we believed she had become a danger to herself. Her actions were not making sense, and she was making bad decisions. While we lived in Florida, we had locals keep an eye on the house and asked them to let us know if she really did return. Unfortunately, we did learn that she was back in the house the morning of the 6th and made the call to APS.

The situation continued to become even more bizarre. Later that day, the facility called me and asked for Louise's phone number. At first, they didn't say why, and when I pressed for why this was needed, I was told "she took your mom out to look at apartments and didn't come back." I was astonished by this as I knew that Mom had been back in her own house for hours. When I made this point, I was asked again for the number as she needed to reach out to Louise "now." I gave her the number. Sure enough, I got a call back a few minutes later. Like **Thelma and Louise** in the movie of the same name, they had made a break for it. They left under false pretenses and the facility let me know that they, too, had been interacting with APS, regarding this turn of events.

Apparently, Louise told the facility representative that she was "astounded" that she was expected to bring her back and that she had no plans to do so. I will never know for sure who said what, or what Louise really believed, but the bottom line is that my mom left the facility without officially being discharged and Louise seemed to believe Mom was more able to be alone than was truly the case. Between Mom and Louise, they created a picture of "reality" that was anything but and set forth on a path that made an already difficult situation infinitely worse. Whether purposefully or not, just doesn't matter. When Mom left, she put her life in danger. She left with no instructions regarding continued medication use, no arrangements made for continuing therapy and assistance, and no help. To our knowledge she had made no arrangements for groceries or other daily needs. So much for taking charge of her discharge planning, as she had said she would.

Once we learned that my mom had not even been properly discharged, we called the local police department and asked them to do a wellness check, since she would not answer the phone, and continued her plan of not speaking to her family. They were at first reluctant to do this, despite the fact that we were concerned for her safety, and we own the house, but eventually agreed. That said, they emphasized that she has the right to do this kind of thing. An officer did go to the house, and she told him she was ok, but she was "mad at her daughter." It was embarrassing to hear this, but just another ugly statement in a long list of them unfortunately. And more importantly, her "ok" status was extremely short-lived.

At 4:25 am on the 7th, less than 18 hours after the great escape, our phone rang. It was the medical alert company that we use, letting us know that Mom's alarm had gone off, they couldn't reach her, and paramedics were enroute. We told them to enter via the backdoor lock box. They immediately transported her to the hospital. **She had not made it 24 hours in the house alone.**

From bad to worse

I called the hospital even before she got there and gave them the background. I let them know that I have Durable Power of Attorney, including for Health. That said when I called back again for an update, I was told "your mother is stable, but she has asked that we give out no additional information."

My husband and I again found ourselves in a situation in which she was expecting to live in a house we own, supported by a medical alert service we pay for, but allowing us no access to updates about her status. She has rights, but what about ours? We called APS again and updated them on this latest turn of events. And when would anyone other than her family look at my mother holistically and consider that the fact that she was making decisions counter to her own best interests might be an indication of a deeper health problem?

We received a call on her second day in the hospital from a social worker who had spoken with my mother. We again repeated all the background that we had given APS, and she said she would file her own APS report. She did seem to agree that my mom was behaving in a way that was a danger to herself, but beyond documenting it, there was little she could do at that point.

Another day passed, and we then received a call from the hospital from a care coordinator saying your "mother is ready to be discharged." We were astonished. Had she not spoken to any of the previous people with whom I've shared her background? What had changed? We were told that she is "alert and orientated (sic)" and she wants to go home. As it turns out, my mother was telling them she had help at home that was nonexistent, that her children whom she'd disowned would pick her up, and overall painted a picture of her home support network that was simply untrue. And ironically, despite their unwillingness to give me updates about her health, I was the first person they called to get her discharged. We were told that if we couldn't make it back to Michigan to take her home, they could arrange for an ambulance service to take her, or possibly Uber or Lyft. There's a big difference between a medical transportation service and these other options, but neither would get her beyond her front door. What then? Right after we hung up with her, we made an appointment with a home care company that had been referred to us by A Place for Mom to discuss some home care options.

My husband and I once again got on a plane to Michigan. On the way to the hospital, we stopped at my mom's house and took photos of what we found there. Louise had gotten her some milk, a loaf of bread, a carton of eggs, and a Whopper hamburger, which was partially eaten. Beyond that, her refrigerator and freezer were empty as we had cleaned them out while she was in rehab since they'd been full of expired and rotten food. She had not set up her medicine tray for the week. She had already thrown garbage in the sink. There was clearly no plan to take care of any of this following her "break-out" from rehab with Louise. What were they thinking?

When we got to the hospital, we were shocked to find her catheterized and she said she had not been out of bed in a while. How is a person who is in bed and catheterized ready for discharge? We were finally able to get a little more insight into what happened that brought her back to the hospital so soon after leaving rehab. She told us that she had a splitting headache while in bed and pressed the medical alert button herself. Sadly, Mom sometimes experienced headaches and nausea resulting from her various medical conditions. This happened several times while she was in the rehab center and was increasing in frequency.

As people came in and out of the room, we tried to locate the care coordinator who had called us to say Mom was ready for discharge. It turns out that she was off that day, but we had the great good fortune to meet a nurse who came to check on Mom. She is the first person in the hospital who put it all together, listened to us, and considered both my mom's physical health, but also what she was saying, the credibility of it, and her best interests. She treated my mom respectfully but made her answer some hard questions. We told her that we are working on home care, but the company said they would need about two weeks to place someone with Mom. Until then, there just wasn't enough help for Mom in her current even more weakened state.

The nurse had physical and occupational therapy come in to check Mom's ability to get up; she told Mom that people on their way out the door of the hospital typically need to be using the bathroom, not a catheter; and make an overall effort themselves to ask to get up and sit in the chair. When the therapists came in, we were horrified to see that Mom could not get out of bed on her own, and while she walked to the door with a walker, the therapists never let go of her. They recommended that she go back to rehab and complete more therapy, as her stint back in the hospital had eroded the progress she'd made in rehab. The nurse asked my mom whether she would commit to this, to taking it seriously, so that she could go back home with a better plan. Aside from being "alert and orientated (sic)" how on earth had she been judged ready to go home alone to her house? Had we not encountered this caring, wonderful nurse, we have no idea what would have happened. We do know that we would not have taken Mom back to her house in that condition.

Because she had left AMA (against medical advice) from the first rehab facility, we needed to find another facility to take her for the estimated two weeks believed necessary to regain her strength. We again reviewed our options and selected the other highly rated facility in her area. Mom did work with us during this plan, and we thought we were making progress on reversing her disownment of her family. She even participated in a Zoom call with the home care company; they wanted her input on what services she needed and the kind of person she'd like them to find to help her. We had a rational discussion about how expensive home care is and how we would need to work together to pay for it. I left for the day feeling relieved and hopeful that we were on a better path.

De ja vu all over again

The next morning, we brought clothes, toiletries, cell phone, Kindle, and other things to make her time in the new rehab facility as comfortable as possible. When we arrived, we found her refusing to cooperate with the staff and all her anger at me had returned in full force. She again accused me of wanting her out of her house. I told her that the opposite was true… and reminded her that she was the one who said that she was getting out. I told her that while I had no choice but to regretfully accept her decision when she cut off all communication with me and my brothers, she was the one who made that decision, not me. I made the point that she'd been getting some very bad advice from Louise and was horrified that she had left her to fend for herself alone. And of course, it seemed to be completely lost on her that I was once again standing in her room trying to help her in spite of the horrible things she continued to say to and about me. I'm grateful to my husband, who also talked to her and supported me.

My husband and I returned to Florida and updated other family members. I kept in touch with the rehab facility about how things were progressing, and the feedback was mixed. She needed extra encouragement to participate and sometimes refused to do so. But I was pleased with the attentiveness of the staff and the extra efforts they took with her. One of them got her to laugh and when she asked Mom who she should work with on her discharge planning, Mom told her, "My bossy daughter Lynda." I took this as progress!

We had a couple of calls focused on making plans to go home. Medicare was firm about the discharge date.

CHAPTER 4

DISCHARGE PLAN –
THE BIG ELEPHANT IN
THE ROOM

On May 23, we had a discharge call focused on finalizing plans for her May 28 discharge. I was relieved to hear that she had made some good progress. She could dress herself and practiced walking up a ramp like she has on the outside of her home. But there was an elephant in the room. I could hear the hesitation in their voice about her "transfer" capabilities – the up and down acts of getting out of chairs, using the bathroom, and getting in and out of bed. This was exactly the same concern voiced by the rehab facility from which she had bolted – and a concern that our entire family has had as we've watched her progress in recent months.

We arranged private home care three days a week, but that leaves a lot of open time. They suggested "we might want to think about increasing that or maybe having family stay with her." My mom chimed in on the call saying, "I'll be fine." So, here we are, once again, living in the gap. Paying for 24/7 home care at $29/hr would cost $254,000/year! (And even if someone will work for half of that, the annual rate is not affordable.) As it stands, even the current plan will clean out Mom's remaining funds and start moving into my husband's and my funds in just a few short months, if the waiver program doesn't kick in. And if you increase the hours, even if that was affordable, how do you pick the right ones? My mom's previous encounters with EMS had typically been in the middle of the night. Do you choose that over having someone during the day to help her with the numerous things that need attending to every day? That seems a poor choice.

Our family is small, Mom's house is small, and identifying some-one available to sleep on her couch indefinitely who doesn't have other life commitments, is also a woman, who also has the physical strength and expertise needed to assist her intimately – we're talking about an impossible situation. I understand that the rehab team needed to voice their concerns. I share them. But my mom had already firmly rejected moving to assisted living, so we're left with everyone doing the best we can and keeping our fingers crossed. There is a lot of talk about the importance of helping the elderly age in their homes, but the reality is that home care options are incredibly expensive, and simply unaffordable to many. Relying on family members (if they exist) to put their own life on hold, to do things that are physically, emotionally, and financially draining, really isn't a good societal plan in general, and may be impossible anyway. But here we are.

The discharge call also shed additional insight into what may have caused my mom to fall ill with that headache so quickly after leaving the last rehab facility against doctor's advice. They went through a detailed list of her medications and the list had grown substantially since she was orig-inally hospitalized. When she left without being properly discharged, she left without getting these additional prescriptions and it seems likely that her body reacted to this disruption. (And of course, it isn't clear whether she took any medication at all once she left.) Additionally, they provided helpful input on the type of walker she needed, and the fact that she must go see her primary care physician within 3-5 days of discharge to get her prescriptions updated. When "Thelma and Louise" did their break-out, none of this was considered. When Mom told her kids that she was taking over her discharge plans from the first facility, apparently, she just meant that she would get a ride somewhere. She made no attempt to actually create a plan or close things out. I've learned that there really is a method to the discharge process madness and Mom ignored this important step and paid a very high price and brought her entire family along for the ride.

Discharge derailed

With the discharge date set for May 28th, I planned to return to Michigan on the 26th to make sure her house was ready, that she had groceries, to get acquainted with her care giver, and to take her to follow-up doctor's appointment. And family members were planning to help as well. Once again, our plans took a hit. Her case manager called the day before my flight with the scary news that she had contracted COVID 19. Although she had been vaccinated and boosted, she was definitely high risk, given her age, diabetes, and several other health factors. And beyond that, I knew that she would take this news hard, and likely her suspicions would return about people plotting to keep her institutionalized.

Sure enough, when I landed, I found a voice mail message from my mom saying that it was time to pick her up. With the help of the staff, we did our best to reassure her that we would pick her up as soon as she completed the isolation period. Fortunately, thanks to her vaccine and booster, her COVID was very mild. Unfortunately, during the period in which her return home was delayed, the care giver who was scheduled to work with my mom took another job and a new search had to be started.

This experience prompted me to recall the prophetic words of someone I was chatting with during Mom's first stay in rehab. They said, "home care is both essential and incredibly unreliable." I want to be clear here to underscore that no one is suggesting that this worker group is somehow filled with low-quality employees. In fact, the opposite is true. But this is a hard job, often at the lower end of the pay scale, with variable and sometimes limited hours. And COVID brought new challenges and strains to everyone in the healthcare/home care realm. These people are saints and deserve respect and better pay given the critical service they provide.

Discharge day arrives

Fortunately, the home care company was able to identify someone who could start once Mom was released. Mom was released on a Friday and this individual was scheduled to start the following Monday. I went to the facility to pick her up, admittedly feeling a lot of trepidation.

Emotionally she wanted to be home, but was she really up to it? When I met with the unit manager to go over her discharge papers, he handed me a document and said, "I need you to sign this." When I asked what I was signing, he said that it's an acknowledgement that "you're responsible for her." The document indicated that she needed regular supervision and one person available to assist with walking and transitions. So once again, the system gets to make pronouncements about what people "should do," and even attempt to hold them accountable while concurrently offering minimal and hard to obtain support. And even more frustrating, my mom had adamantly refused to accept the assisted living option which would have provided this kind of 24/7 attention, saying cruel things to me in the process, yet I am the one who is responsible for making her preferred option work? There is something very wrong with this picture. Nevertheless, I signed the document as I really don't blame the facility or the unit manager. I think they did their best amid a difficult situation but I'm flagging this as a tangible illustration of what living in the gap really means. It's the classic "darned if you do, darned if you don't" situation.

It took two strong young men to get her settled into my car. One of them looked me over and candidly said, "you are not going to be able to get her out of this car and into the house by yourself." I told him he was absolutely right and that my sister-in-law was waiting at Mom's house for us to arrive. Following the short drive home, we did manage to get her out of the car, up the ramp and into the house, but it was a struggle. Mom was exhausted and settled into her favorite chair while my sister-in-law and I set about making sure that we clearly understood her medication schedule and putting away and washing the clothes she had in rehab. We set up her "pill tray" for a month and it took both of us – two reasonably intelligent people – nearly two hours to go through her discharge papers and care guidelines in the process. Our experience put a further spotlight on the folly of the Thelma and Louise break-out from the first facility. While my mom ultimately is most culpable for leaving without a discharge plan, my anger at Louise for leaving Mom in a clearly untenable situation remains. An already bad situation could have been much worse, even tragic.

CHAPTER 5

REALITY OF LIFE
BACK AT HOME

That first day did little to ease my concerns about the viability of her being alone. I slept uneasily on the couch surrounded by dueling clocks cuckooing and chiming through the night. It was a huge relief to make it to morning and then to reach the 24 hours-at-home point. Mom was exhausted and limited her movement to the bathroom and going to bed. Although the kitchen was only a few feet away from her favorite chair, it might as well have been on the moon. She was conserving her strength for exhausting and essential trips to the bathroom.

I remained in town for the first few days and met with the visiting nurse who helped assess the services that would be needed at home. I also met with the home care aide who would be coming three times a week. Mom was not happy about the prospect of these people coming in. "I don't want all of these people coming in my house." I did my best to highlight the value that they bring and the point that overall, the amount of time people would be there was fairly minimal in the overall scheme of things. And I was blunt. While the nurse, physical therapist, and occupational therapist would likely only come for a few weeks, the three times per week home care aide was essential on a permanent basis. Her bossy daughter surfaced, and I told her that point was non-negotiable. I arranged for these people to call me to set up appointments to help ensure that the services were delivered and that she did not cancel them as she has done in the past.

During those first few days, I reminded her about her medications and ensured that she had meals. I was worried that she wasn't drinking enough fluids. She told me that they had given her that feedback in the hospital as well. Although forgetting the things Mom had said to me over the previous few weeks will never be in the cards, we were able to reconnect a bit and have more "normal" interactions. Most of the time, she seemed to be tracking pretty well, but then moments arose like her question, "do I have a cat? I thought I had a cat." I reminded her that she did have a cat, but we'd moved it to my daughter's house while she was in rehab. We had actually discussed that previously and she was very relieved at the time, but the entire plan seemed to have been forgotten, including the name of the cat.

The rehab facility had told us that she should not return to using her 4-wheel walker but should use a 2-wheel walker instead. That made good sense because they were fearful that the 4-wheel walker would get away from her. The challenge with that was that the 4-wheel walker had a seat that she used to sit on when she went to the kitchen, and she also used the seat as a tray when she went from room-to-room. I did some research and found a lightweight tray that fit over the handles of the 2-wheel walker. She couldn't sit on it, of course, but it did help a bit logistically. Nevertheless, changing something like a walker can actually be a huge factor in an individual's day-to-day life experiences. The more a caregiver can anticipate the moves that need to be made, the better able they will be able to figure out how to help. Making sure that critical items are within easy reach is also very important.

One area of significant concern for me was self-care like bathing, shampooing hair, cutting nails, and the like. Obviously, the ability to do these things is a key daily life ingredient, and they are private, personal activities. This has been an area of struggle for Mom for some time, but she absolutely would not acknowledge it or accept home help with these activities. I understand why this is sensitive and embarrassing, for sure. At the same time, one needs to do these things. She continued to maintain that she was handling these things herself and refused an available option for help with these functions. She got mad at me when I suggested it and though I brought it up reluctantly on more than one occasion, she continued to say that she didn't need any help. We installed an emergency button in the shower and ensured lots of towels are on-hand but worry that this is not really a good solution.

For meals, we came up with a plan for the home care worker to create meals while she was there. I've also looked for things that are very simple and pre-packaged for times when she was by herself. For example, "Lunchables" that my granddaughters have for lunch were actually well-received by Mom. While processed foods are not ideal, I concluded things like that that include a bit of meat and cheese are better than just eating junk food and candy. I've also been in touch with Meals on Wheels. They have a waiting list and we joined it. Of course, Mom said, "I've heard those meals aren't good." Turns out her feedback came from my grandmother who has been dead for 28 years! For my part, I'm grateful for services like Meals on Wheels!

After a few days, it was time for me to return to my home in Florida. I was hopeful that Mom would make it at least 60 days in her home, in order to fulfill the Medicare benefit period requirements. This distance was increasingly problematic and, while I won't digress too far beyond the overall theme of this story, I will say that by June 2022, my husband and I made the decision to leave Florida and move back to Michigan. The result was that on top of dealing with all of the challenges in Michigan, we added a move into the mix, with all that entails. But something had to give. I wrapped up a business project in April, continuing to face constant expensive travel back and forth between Michigan and Florida, along with complex issues that are too difficult to navigate long-distance. Our own vision and plans for retirement had been completely derailed and it was time to regroup.

Once back in Florida, I began receiving calls from the nurse, the physical therapist, and occupational therapist about appointments. They would call me and then I would call Mom and let her know when to expect visits. This worked for a few days, but then the nastiness returned. She said she didn't want these people in her house, that they were a waste of money, they don't really do anything, and she was going to keep the blinds closed so they can't tell she's home. She told me to cancel the services.

She also told other relatives that she had told me to do this. These relatives then contacted me to express their concern about her not getting the service. So essentially, I was getting it from all sides. Mom was complaining about the services and other family was telling me that Mom really needs the services – as if I didn't know that!

I told her that I wasn't comfortable cancelling after she'd only been home a couple of weeks. I called the company, and we calibrated the services somewhat, so that one fewer person would be coming. That plan continued for a couple more weeks, at which point she began denying access to care providers when they arrived or saying that she had forgotten about the appointments. I had one poor woman call me from outside my mother's house, worried because the blinds were closed, and no one was answering the door. She feared that my mother was ill or incapacitated within. I called Mom and she immediately picked up and said she was fine; she just didn't want to do the physical therapy. It was disappointing that she seemed ok with letting another human being waste their own time and worry about her as well. I called the therapist back, explained the situation, and apologized for wasting her time. Ultimately Mom cancelled everything but the three-day per week care provider. At least I succeeded in making it clear to both my mom and that provider's company, that cancelling that service was not an option. And the even better news there was that Mom came to enjoy having this caregiver three days a week. One day she told me "she keeps me organized," very high praise indeed, coming from Mom. Again, the referral to this company came from "A Place for Mom;" and I'm grateful to this agency and "A Place for Mom" for their help.

Spending out of control

Once she was home, I began keeping an eye on Mom's bills and her credit card spending again. I also did her grocery shopping via Instacart, which gave me additional insight into how things were going. Alarm bells began happening with increasing frequency. Mom loves Red Rose Tea. I was surprised when my sister-in-law sent me a text on Mom's behalf, asking me to add Red Rose Tea to her next grocery order, as I was sure she had at least two large boxes on-hand. Nevertheless, I ordered an extra box just in case I was misremembering that. A few days later, I noticed a number of large Amazon charges had been made. In addition to other items, she had ordered large quantities of Red Rose Tea bags as well as pods. During my July visits to Michigan, I found that she had enough tea on hand to serve tea to several large banquet halls. Not only can she not afford this, but her purchases were beginning to encroach on space in her small home. Giant bags of popcorn, candy, shoes, purses, were all consuming her money and space. And of course, some of these things are anything but healthy to eat. Let me be clear, I am guilty of eating things I shouldn't as well, and don't begrudge my mother things that please her, but the financial, space, and health impacts of these purchases when taken together were alarming and potentially harmful on multiple fronts.

Seeing a purchase of a new Kindle for $160 raised the concerns to a new level. I discussed this with her when I was in Michigan to try to understand what was driving the purchase. This new Kindle was inferior to the one she already had. She did not know how to set it up and didn't purchase essential accessories. She said she ordered it because her current Kindle wasn't bright enough but later realized that she didn't need it after she ordered it when the "brightness returned" to her original Kindle. I set the new one up for her as an extra back-up (she already has a back-up Kindle and an iPad) but my worry about her purchasing habits grew even more. My hope was that moving back to Michigan would help me stay ahead of these things more effectively.

Thelma and Louise – Post Break-out

Upon returning home, my mom was looking forward to returning to those nightly calls with Louise. While they had spoken every day when she was in the first nursing home, that did not continue during the hospitalization after her "break-out" and second rehab facility stay. I know that Louise was having some medical issues of her own, including a surgery, and I suppose it is also possible that her children may have discouraged the calls given her role in the break-out debacle. I just don't know. Whatever the reason, my mom missed the calls and hoped to reconnect when she was home. While I had my own misgivings about the relationship, I knew it was important to my mom, and let Louise's daughter know that Mom was home, but left it for them to take it from there.

That said, she was not able to rekindle the camaraderie and close relationship that made the calls so enjoyable for her. She told me that Louise seemed reluctant to talk when she called. Mom attributed this to Louise's medical issues and need to recover from her surgery, and that may very well be the case. While Louise's influence on my mother, and the downstream damage that has been done to my family as a result has been profound, and I had no interest in speaking with her myself, it saddened me to see my mother missing someone who has been so important to her. And I can't help but wish I believed that she valued her own family in a similar way. Sadly, my mom has always expected her children to take the initiative to call and visit her, rarely reaching out to call any of us on her own "just because."

CHAPTER 6

IT FALLS
APART AGAIN

I visited Michigan twice in July 2022 and then the plan was that I would not return until we officially moved at the end of August. That would leave a few weeks between visits, but I had work to do in Florida to get ready for the move. On the positive side, Mom connected well with the caregiver who came three days a week, and I know appreciated her help. She was attentive to Mom, but twelve hours a week leaves a lot of alone time. So, I was worried about being away that long.

Turns out that my fears were valid. We had two incidents with her handling of the phone. When it isn't hung up properly, it loses its charge, and then she is unreachable. And she is notorious for not answering the phone even in the best of times. The caller ID would show up on her TV screen and she told me often that so and so had called but she didn't feel like talking to them. And even though we gave her a cell phone for emergencies, she rarely answered or used that either. I did my best to be clear that she needed to answer all of my calls. Anyway, I had to call others twice in the course of a week and ask them to go over to check on her because I couldn't reach her. They hung up the phone so it would recharge and reported back that she was ok, but this was another illustration of how things were just not in a good place.

Then on August 5, a little over 60 days from when she had returned home, my husband and I were celebrating our 44th anniversary with dinner at home in Florida amidst all the packing boxes, when I got a call from my sister-in-law. She had stopped by Mom's house to visit and found her lethargic and not tracking well. She also had Twinkies in her lap that she had apparently intended to eat but had not done so. We concluded that a call to EMS was in order. They quickly arrived and I stayed on the line. It turns out that her sugar was very low, and they treated her there and got her stabilized. They said that they figured that she could feel her sugar dropping and grabbed the Twinkies in an effort to feel better. They read her the riot act (nicely) about her eating habits and the downside of processed food and then left. My wonderful sister-in-law stayed the night to keep an eye on her and I got a flight to Michigan. So much for not returning until the end of August. I was returning only three weeks after my last visit.

In the morning, Mom was still pretty weak and when she tried to get out of bed, slid to the floor. My sister-in-law was unable to help her up and again needed to call EMS. I learned about this second call when I picked up my voice mail after my flight landed. They got her up and back into bed and my sister-in-law told me that she stayed in bed until just before I arrived at her house.

When I got there, she had made it out to the living room but hadn't eaten much and was complaining of a headache. We tried to get her to eat and made sure she took her medication and I continued to encourage her to eat after my sister-in-law left. I asked her whether she needed to go to the bathroom several times and made the point that it was essential that she eat and be able to get up and move around a bit. She had difficulty taking even small bites and when she tried to get up, she was unable to do so. There was no way I could leave her in this condition.

After several attempts it was obvious that she could not get out of the chair, and I was unable to help her reach a standing position by myself. By that point, she was desperate to go to the bathroom, so I called my brother to see if he was around to help. He came right over, and it took both of us to get her out of the chair. The bathroom then became a new, and embarrassing frontier for all three of us as we helped her get situated there. **I cannot overstate the physical difficulty we experienced**. Even together, my brother and I could not effectively handle moving her.

Once she was ready to leave the bathroom, she concluded that going back to the living room was not possible and wanted to go to her bed. This was also difficult, and even though my brother and I worked to help her, we could not get her properly situated on the bed. She was continuing to struggle keeping food and fluids down, so I called EMS for the third time in 24 hours and said that, despite her own desire to stay home, I thought she needed to go to the hospital.

They agreed that she needed to go and loaded her in the ambulance. I cannot say enough about the EMS services. They joked with my mom and said they know they're extremely handsome, but gently made the point that calling EMS three times in 24 hours is not the best plan and she needs to take care of herself. I went to the emergency room with her. It turns out that in addition to very low blood sugar again, she was dehydrated. I stayed with her until they said she would need to be admitted, and then left for the night, as it was quite late by then, and I try to avoid driving in the dark.

I had scheduled a return to Florida to wrap up packing and wanted to understand what the next steps for Mom were going to need to be, so spent a lot of time in the hospital with her. She was completely bedridden for two days, after which the physical therapist and occupational therapist came to evaluate her. She could not get out of bed without help and was only able to take a few short steps sideways. They got her up and sitting in a chair for an hour at a time and concluded that rehab would once again be necessary.

She seemed to understand that going home was not immediately viable, although still voiced that desire constantly. She also asked that I order a lift chair to help her get out of the chair in the living room, as her last experience at home trying to get up had clearly made an impression on her. I started looking into chair options, but also worried that a new chair won't help with the bathroom or getting in and out of bed. I made the arrangements for her to go to rehab again and let the home care agency know that she would not need help for some period of time. This worried me as Mom had been so comfortable with the person who has been coming to the house, and it was likely she would need to be reassigned.

And the dehydration diagnosis highlighted another one of those pesky elephants in the room. We all constantly reminded her about the importance of drinking fluids for a variety of reasons. We make sure she has easy access to water, milk, and juice, as well as the tea she loves. (It's important to remember that the caffeine in tea can increase dehydration.) Her care giver pre-opened bottles for her to use when she was by herself. She always acknowledged that she should drink more but continued to limit her intake. My theory is that she does this to minimize the number of times she has to get up to go to the bathroom, because that is so painful to her knees, and it helps her deal with her incontinence. She doesn't want to discuss any of this and says she will drink more, but here we are.

And maybe the biggest elephant in the room of all is this…it seems clear that if my sister-in-law hadn't dropped in that Friday night, chances were high that the combination of dehydration and low blood sugar could have created an even more serious and potentially even fatal outcome. Despite her intense desire to be at home, without 24-hour care, the risks were clearly increasing, not dissipating.

Although Mom had a home health aide, all of these issues occurred on the weekend, when the aide is not scheduled to work. When my sister-in-law and I talked about the challenge of figuring out the "right hours" to have help available, she made the point that the best times would be when the cared-for individual needs to get up or down. Never were truer words spoken. Of course, that sort of ad hoc schedule is impossible in a home environment but is why assisted living or nursing home care is so useful. And this is when all of the financial models come roaring back to bite the elderly. Once my mom's remaining funds were spent on the home care she uses, the plan was to apply for a special program in Michigan aimed at keeping people in their homes. What was unknown at this point is the extent to which this can help, and whether returning home would even be viable given her current condition. We were back to just taking it one-day-at-a-time.

CHAPTER 7

REHAB REDUX

Mom returned to the rehab facility that she had left a couple of months back, and the staff began working with her again. It is a nice place, with each person having their own room and bathroom. I brought in clothes and her Kindle, but when I asked her if she wanted anything from home to include in the room, she said "no, I'm not staying here very long." Family members brought flowers and magazines, but the room remained kind of bare.

While a desire to leave is an important ingredient to actually going home, that needs to be supported by genuine effort and progress in achieving the physical capabilities to do that. Once again, Mom's participation in physical therapy was kind of half-hearted. Just as in the past, the staff continuously made the point to her that she needs to take ownership for getting up and participating, acknowledging that this is very hard work and painful. That said, she would sometimes decline, saying she didn't feel like it. She would tell me that "I'll do whatever they tell me," but rarely pushed to get involved or set goals for herself. Instead, she would tell me things like "they didn't have time to work with me," or "I don't want to bother anyone," subtle ways to push the responsibility elsewhere. And because the therapy is painful, she claimed that it was making her worse. And who am I to say it wasn't? Perhaps the pain was exhausting her and making her weaker. Regardless of the real reason, her progress in being able to get around was hard to see.

Her interest in food diminished and she complained constantly about the meals she was served, pushing them away the moment they arrived. I have to say that the food looked great to me! That said, we reminded her that she can request alternative options 24 hours a day, and did that on her behalf at times, but this became a new area of concern. When I tried to talk about eating as another piece of the puzzle to help get stronger, she told me she just feels like punching people who say things like that. While the comment lacked the venom she'd directed at me in the past, I was bummed that the idea of punching me remained on her mind. The anger at her situation was still bubbling under the surface.

The one thing she continued to talk about was getting a lift chair to help get out of her chair at home. We looked at them together and selected one that I then ordered for her so that the house would be ready. I hoped that this might encourage her to keep her head in the game and work on the things she needed to do to return home. The downside is that a lift chair doesn't help with bathroom visits or getting in and out of bed, and other transitions that need to happen. And experts warn that over-use of the chair as a substitute for using one's own muscles can actually be counterproductive. We did discuss these points, but I don't think that she really took them to heart.

After about a month, her progress in getting up and down was still inconsistent. She talked even more about going home while her willingness to eat decreased. She often refused food as it arrived, saying it was "terrible." (The food always looked fine.) The dietician called me to discuss this, noting that Mom was losing weight, and said that she would work on getting more of the simple sandwiches and snack-type items my mom liked into her menu plan, with the hope that she would eat a little more. Mom did tell me one day "I figure if I don't eat the food here, they'll let me go home." This provided a little insight into her strategy. I tried unsuccessfully to talk about this once again, noting that food and the associated calories help give her energy, that they help her with mobility, and that these are the things that need to come together in order to go home. This strategy of not eating wasn't helping her, but no one was able to convince her. They did start bringing her different things, but she refused the new items as well.

She said endlessly that "I just want to go home and sit in my chair." Every time she said that I said I'd like that too, but it's important to be able to navigate getting to the bathroom and to bed, that sitting in her chair exclusively isn't really an option. Sometimes she'd acknowledge that was a good point, and other times she said she was sure she would have no problem getting around, even though she was clearly having trouble with mobility. She was not even able to sit up or move herself without help within her bed, so it was hard to see how things could work at home.

One day when I came in, she said she was ready to go and indicated that someone (she wasn't sure who) had told her she was going home that day. I was surprised to hear this. I went to the nurses' station to inquire as I would have expected a call if true, and indeed, there was no current discharge date scheduled. When I told Mom that, she was very upset. I am not sure how she came to think this, whether there was a misunderstanding, or that she was just wishing it so hard that she determined that the day had arrived. I tried to explain about the discharge planning process, but I don't think I connected.

She stepped up her campaign to leave by refusing participation in physical therapy. The day arrived when a member of the PT team asked me to step out into the hall for a chat when I was visiting. She told me that Mom had told her outright that she was going to be nasty so that "you'll let me out." She said that Mom was not being productive in PT and had even taken to being unhelpful, and staying limp, when they tried to move her, resulting in the staff needing to exert more energy, and do more work, in their efforts to get her up. She indicated that she wanted to give me a heads up that this would likely result in her discharge. The staff member's words were prophetic, as later that day the caseworker called me to say that after consulting with Medicare, Mom's discharge date had been set to occur the following week.

This call put my anxiety through the roof. I had trouble getting my head around how a woman who wasn't eating, and whose poor eating habits were a key driver for her most recent hospitalization, and whose mobility issues seemed to be increasing (at least to my eyes), was ready to go home. But I can also see the logic of discharging someone from a rehab facility who refuses to participate in rehab!

Not only was I concerned about the physical realities of keeping her safe, but my concerns about her financial viability accelerated. Her small banking account was dwindling while her credit card balance kept increasing. I did immediately call the caregiver who had been working with us prior to her hospitalization and was relieved that she could return to work with Mom. That said, I was extremely worried about the limited schedule and whether it would be enough. I resolved to discuss this in more detail during the discharge planning meeting that had been scheduled, as well as to have some conversations with Mom (again) about the things she needs to do to keep safe.

Another discharge planning meeting

Things took a turn at the discharge planning meeting. The staff walked through Mom's progress and indicated that she was not only not improving, but her ability to get up and down was regressing. They said she was getting weaker and that it required two people to move her. (This was consistent with what my brother and I had experienced.) It was abundantly clear that going home supported by a home health aide three days a week was simply not going to work. This experience put a special spotlight for me on the word "discharge." When a rehab facility says that Medicare has directed it's time to discharge someone, that doesn't necessarily mean discharge to home. It can also mean that the individual is considered to no longer be in a position to benefit from rehab therapy and therefore must leave. And that was the case with my mom. While she had managed to go home from this same facility a few months ago, that was not in the cards now. So, unlike the previous times where there some equivocation, this time there was none. Not only did she not have two people at home around to help, but she also didn't even have one consistently. There was no way we could provide what she needed at home. So, my own assessment was actually pretty accurate and my fears about her going home well-founded.

That said, she only wanted to go home, there was nothing else on her mind. We'd finally hit the point Mom had been dreading and we did our best to explain that to her. She asked if she could just "try going home for a week." It was a difficult conversation because it was clear that going home wasn't possible and the next step needed to be long-term care. Her caseworker made a referral to a nearby long-term care facility that had Medicaid availability and my husband and I went there to tour and to talk about the admissions process, including the steps we needed to take to apply for Medicaid.

They were friendly and helpful, and we worked with the administration on the paperwork and scheduled an admissions date. We let other family members know about the plan. My sister-in-law visited my mom the next day and let me know that Mom didn't seem to know she was not going home. Apparently, our discussion with the care team had not really registered. So, I went back to talk to her about it again, reviewing the key points of the meeting, and why it wouldn't work to go home. I told her I would meet her at the new place as a medical transport company would be giving her a ride. She was disappointed but didn't argue that she could handle things on her own at home.

CHAPTER 8

LONG-TERM CARE BEGINS

Mom moved into the long-term care facility on a Friday. We did our best to get her room set-up with a TV, her clothes, and her beloved Red Rose Tea. We brought a picture of my dad to hang on the wall, and she asked if we could get a bigger one. I did manage to blow up the photo, although the resolution was not optimal. I was very relieved when she said that the people there were nice! And I was pleased to see that she was out-of-bed and dressed when I visited. That said, she still wasn't eating much.

A few days after she arrived, I came in one morning and found her still in bed. She said she wasn't feeling very well and seemed very tired. As we were talking, the right side of her mouth started drooping and her words became garbled. I was alarmed that she might be having a stroke and quickly got the staff to check her. They called for an ambulance to get her to the hospital. I followed in my car and met her in the emergency room.

They asked her all sorts of questions and she was pretty confused. She didn't know the year, the month, or why she was there. When asked for my name, she provided her own. Twice that day she said the year was 1988. When I went home that night I thought about that year and had a possible ah-ha moment. 1988 was the year before my mom and dad moved to Florida; this was something dad wanted to do, but Mom was not as enthusiastic about it. My younger sister moved with them, but the rest of Mom's family and friends remained in Michigan. Mom and my sister were very close, and Mom was devastated when my sister died in childbirth in Florida at the very young age of 37. I can't help but wonder if among Mom's musings as she sat alone in her favorite chair at home was the "what if" game….what if they hadn't moved to Florida? Would my sister still be alive? This is just a theory as Mom would never really talk about this kind of thing, but it does provide a plausible explanation for why Mom seemed stuck in 1988 for a while.

I told her I loved her when I left that day, and she said she loved me too. I'm not sure who she really had in mind when she said that, but it was nice to hear, nevertheless.

The conclusion was that she had not had a stroke, but more likely a TIA, transient ischemic attack, that behaves like a stroke, but typically lasts only a little while before symptoms resolve. They admitted her for observation and once again, physical therapy was recommended for her when she returned to her long-term care center. The physical therapist turned out to be someone whom I had encountered a few months back when Mom was in that hospital for her pot roast injury. The point was made that, although very weak, she still had strength that could be used to make improvements in mobility, but of course, a big piece of this was dependent upon her own motivation and tolerance for the work. And the pain in her bad knee continued to be a powerful motivational detractor as she continued to say that physical therapy just makes her feel worse. I was once again given a copy of exercises she could do herself and I showed it to her, but I knew she wasn't going to do the exercises. By this point, I'd lost track of the number of physical therapists who have tried to help. I know that Mom simply didn't believe in the value of this work and the notion that a little bit of daily effort could make a difference. And who knows? Perhaps because the pain was so intense, it really was making her worse. The only thing that was certain, was that her mobility was severely limited.

I spoke with the doctor and staff about the fact that she wasn't eating, and they decided to try a soft diet. This did not seem to entice her either. While sitting with her for lunch, she ate only two bites of mashed potatoes. During that same lunch, she talked about how all she wants is to "go home and sit in my chair." I tried again to speak about her overall weakness and that she just can't be alone without help and that food is a really important ingredient in being stronger but wasn't able to get her to eat anything more.

Concurrent with keeping an eye on how she was doing at the hospital, I also had to stay in close touch with the long-term care facility as she had just moved there, and I didn't want to lose her space. We were in the middle of the Medicaid application process and were private pay until she reached the asset level at which one can utilize Medicaid. Beyond that, I was also beginning the process of transitioning some of the services she was receiving at her house, as we began getting ready for the eventuality of selling it. Keeping phone, cable, and Internet active in a house no one is in just makes no financial sense.

We decided to give it a little time before taking that step, but we couldn't keep a house that no one is using indefinitely either. The house was so important to her that I worried about her reaction to news of an impending sale.

After a few days in the hospital, she returned to the long-term care facility. Although her speech was a little clearer, she was still struggling a bit with putting her thoughts together. I noticed that some of the updates I had been giving her about family members were not really sticking. She continued to enjoy her Kindle, but I felt bad about her television situation. The TV we got required use of two remotes, one for the cable and one for the TV itself. They also had an option to hook into the facility's Wi-Fi, but she was not able to navigate that either. We did our best to make sure it was turned on to her favorite shows when we visited, but it wasn't ideal.

I arrived one morning to find her working with a physical therapist who was having her do in-bed exercises and encouraging her to work on building her strength so that she could get back out of bed. She cooperated with the therapist, but when she left, she turned to me and said, "I never believed I'd have to be in a place like this." It was a sad moment. Obviously, I wouldn't have chosen this for her – or anyone, for that matter – as the whole concept of privacy and autonomy is compromised. A family member said, "I don't see the big deal; she can still do what she was doing at home – read and watch TV." While that's true, there are other intangible freedoms that we take for granted…the freedom to grab a snack, the freedom to stay in your PJs all day with nobody bugging you to get up and get dressed, and just the peace of being by yourself. Since my dad died, Mom had gotten used to living alone, and liked it. Now she had a chatty roommate, who liked to loudly play the radio. I understood what she was missing, but I was powerless to provide it for her. Ultimately her preferred path was no longer something navigable for her or for her family. We had finally hit the wall and were out of options.

One of the biggest issues continued to be the pain in the leg for which she had not had a knee replacement done. The decision she'd made not to do the second knee replacement seemed to be on her mind more, but she also felt that she had made the right choice at the time. My dad had been very agitated and upset by her hospitalization and the follow-up therapy that she needed for the first knee. And the therapy process on that knee was very painful. She had concluded that it would be simpler for all concerned not to do the second knee.

That decision, along with a separate decision she made to decline a procedure her doctor recommended for another health issue, over time likely led to her increased mobility issues. This reality, along with many "what ifs" about what if she'd been more active, taken a different approach to diet and exercise, rattled around in my mind. But to what end? I could not make her better. And trying to find something or someone to blame serves no purpose. That said, I did make a personal commitment to myself and to my family to do my best to stay active and engaged and take ownership of my own path forward and to try to remain mindful of how my decisions could impact my own future or that of my family. There are no guarantees, and I understand that life takes twists and turns that are out of our control, but that old saying about the importance of focusing on those things that you can control and making the best of those things resonates for me now more than ever. It's especially sad, frustrating, and heartbreaking when you see someone you love suffering when it's quite possible that the act of making different decisions might have minimized or avoided the pain, or even assured their more active participation in life as they wished to live it.

As the days marched on, we did what we could to make Mom's room pleasant and to visit often, but I know she was discouraged. She still said she wanted to go home but started adding, "and if I can't then I want to be kaput" and variations thereof. I dreaded the looming conversation about selling the house and some suggested just not telling her. This was tempting but it just didn't seem respectful to me, and it seemed particularly problematic because it would in essence be doing the exact thing she had once accused me of wanting to do behind her back. And I feared that not telling her could also backfire spectacularly if someone inadvertently mentioned it. For example, people at the facility are referred to as residents. And perhaps she would want to direct a preference for handling certain of her belongings. I didn't think so but couldn't be sure. I concluded honesty would be the best policy and resolved to discuss it with her before we actually listed the house.

However, as the weeks progressed, we began to see more episodes of confusion, and she even talked about her own confusion at times. I had hung a picture of my dad so that she could easily see it, and she would talk about how he had left her first. I said that was true but suggested that he was still keeping an eye on her. She seemed to like that point and agreed. Unfortunately, the confusion increased, and we also began to see her become combative and visibly angry and suspicious of others. They continued to try to do light physical therapy with her (usually bedside) but this was painful, and she accused the staff of being mean and rough.

Her unwillingness to eat and tendency to drink too little, also continued. This resulted in dehydration, which then required that she receive fluids intravenously. This became a merry-go-round in which she would require this IV support periodically.

The combativeness waned, but the confusion began to move to a new level, within which Mom began describing events that didn't happen. At times she thought she was in other locations, or that people had told her things that had not happened, that she'd won the lottery (a lifelong dream), and even that my dad had spoken to her. All of this was incredibly sad. Sometimes this would go on for an entire visit while other times she would interact with us normally. This seemed to suggest that perhaps the disownment of her family that she declared months earlier, may have been driven by some kind of early dementia, rather than her genuine feelings, but we will never know for certain.

While I had hoped to have a conversation with her about the need to sell the house and talk through what she would like to do with her belongings, this was not viable.

The day came, as we were decorating her room for Christmas, when she again said to me, "I never thought I'd be in a place like this," but those words were followed by something different than she'd said in the past. Tears came to my eyes as she went on to say, "but I'm comfortable here." I didn't know then if that sentiment would hold but she said she knows she is safer there than she would be on her own. I concurred, noting that I understood that being there would not be anyone's first choice, but reiterating that it was good to have other people around all the time, and that it was still possible to do many of the things she did at home – watch TV, read her Kindle, listen to the radio, put up Christmas decorations, and visit with family.

Given her treatment of family members in previous months, there were some who were reluctant to visit her again. We had to have "grandma really didn't mean it" conversations with some and let others know that she didn't seem to remember some of her past pronouncements. Ensuring no regrets and finding a way to put some of those difficulties aside seemed to be the best thing to do. Her whole family stood by her.

We carried on with the cycle of good days, bad days, confusion, clarity now being part of our lives. Her interest in food was almost nonexistent and she began experiencing increased episodes of nausea. Family members brought her special treats, and one caring aide even brought her some of her favorites from area restaurants, but she never took more than a couple of bites. The nursing staff worked to mitigate her nausea and vomiting with medication, but I know she was miserable.

Hospice begins

During a care conference in January 2023, we discussed the increased confusion, continuing weight loss, and the difficulty Mom was having with taking her many medications. It was during that meeting that the staff introduced the notion that it might be time for hospice. This would be a way to put the focus more on keeping Mom comfortable by adjusting medications and providing some additional individual help and attention each day. The services included extra nursing help, a daily aide, and visits from a chaplain and social worker.

This seemed like a good idea. We set up the hospice service in mid-January and I'm grateful to say that this did seem to help dissipate her episodes of extreme nausea as they calibrated her medications. That said, her lack of interest in eating continued and her mobility challenges became more pronounced. She was encouraged to get out of bed and get dressed each day, but she often resisted, saying she was just more comfortable in bed.

She grew weaker and weaker, and she spent more time sleeping. When she spoke, it was hard to hear her, as her voice became faint. I tried to keep her current on the latest with family members and was thankful for Facebook, as it provided a way for me to show her pictures of her grandchildren and great-grandchildren at school events and dances. One of my nieces got a new puppy and posted loads of photos that gave my mom great pleasure to see. She had always loved dogs. We kept fresh flowers in her room, especially carnations, hoping that they would provide a little enjoyment.

But I know she spent a lot of time with her own thoughts as she stopped reading her Kindle and lost interest in the radio and television. The hospice team was kind to her. Sometimes she seemed receptive to chatting with them, and other times she just wouldn't engage. There were times that she would tell me that she didn't feel well, but then she would tell the staff she felt ok, so this made it hard for them to know when she needed pain meds.

On February 27, our visit was especially sad. Mom knew we were there but said almost nothing. I gave her some good news about some medical tests that one of her granddaughters had undergone and she mouthed "that's good." I'm so glad she was able to hear and understand this news on what turned out to be her last day with us.

The next morning, at 7:30 am, one of the nurses called to tell me that Mom had passed away. Mom's final journey had been long and painful and incredibly difficult for her and her family. I was grateful to the staff at the nursing facility and the hospice team for their support and could only hope that Mom was now at peace after her long, painful journey.

CHAPTER 9

DEPRESSION? DEMENTIA? COGNITIVE CAPABILITIES?

One of the most common questions I heard from family and friends had to do with Mom's cognitive abilities. People (including me) wanted to be able to explain and understand the reasons behind her meanness and the poor decisions that began occurring. I was regularly asked whether I thought she was depressed or perhaps was suffering from dementia.

I can say that, for months, the staff in the hospitals and rehab facilities generally did not seem to question those abilities. While this did change over time, she was overall coherent and could answer questions they asked. I observed Mom being asked the standard questions…your name is, and birthdate is…the year is…the day of the week is…followed by questions about how she takes care of bathing, cooking, and so on. While some of these questions are verifiable, many are not, and when the respondent is not truthful or claims skills they do not have, the person asking the questions really has no way to know the difference.

What they couldn't see to the same extent as her family were the inconsistencies and even false statements that she made. She said a lot of things that were simply not true but was that due to a cognitive gap or, perhaps more pragmatically in her mind, a desire to achieve a certain result? Maybe a bit of both was going on, there's no way to be sure. To my mind, this was a major area of challenge related to living in this service gap. People in hospitals and nursing centers are very busy and if someone is making statements that sound credible, how are they to know when they're not? When someone tells you that they have help at home, or they live with their son, that they take their own showers, and cook their own meals, how are they to know when that's not the case? Sure, there are occasional conferences with family and daily opportunities for family and staff to compare notes, but there are many, many staff members involved and connecting the dots is incredibly difficult.

She complained that others were taking control of her life, while simultaneously doing very little to engage herself. "You can do it. I don't know how to do that" was a common refrain for a long time, accompanied later with the odious "after all I've done for you, you should do this." This could apply to any of the hundreds of things people need to do to exist. Over the last several years, she rarely left her home and had very limited movement within the home. She watched a lot of TV and read and little else. I know that she had expected my late younger sister to be with her during her final years and really never recovered her equilibrium after we lost her. She spoke about the unfairness of losing my dad when other women she knew still had their husbands. At the risk of sounding like an armchair psychologist, my sense was that she had never managed to move beyond the anger phase in the five stages of grief after losing my dad and my sister. And she absolutely would not talk about anything involving emotions or how she felt about things.

I can appreciate the stress she was undoubtedly feeling as she found herself unable to do basic things on her own while likely contemplating the scary unknowns ahead. I did my best to remain empathetic and let many of her words "go in one ear and out the other," but that didn't make it any easier to deal with the day-to-day realities of trying to help her. I was literally in the world of "darned if I do, darned if I don't." It had happened gradually over a period of many years, but there we were.

As time went on, the overt anger began to be replaced by confusion, lethargy, and sadness. The staff included questions in their regular assessments intended to determine if someone is depressed, including: are you depressed, do you feel like harming yourself, and so on. My mom answered all such questions with an emphatic "NO." I'm not sure how effective this type of assessment is for other people, but for an intensely private person like my mom, I think the chances of her answering honestly are just about nil. And unfortunately, I think it likely that she actually was depressed, but other than trying to spend time with her and talk, I couldn't solve that for her either.

As someone who has always prided myself on problem solving and issue resolution, a sense of failure became a constant companion. I could no longer fulfill my mother's housing expectations and was a regular witness to her physical and emotional pain. I sure couldn't make her better. If I had a magic wand, I would have gladly waved it so she could stay in her house for the rest of her life, with no mobility issues, but I have no magic wand. I did my best, but always felt like I was "a day late and a dollar short," as my dad used to say.

All of this said, the day arrived in which Mom was tested and deemed no longer capable of making her own decisions. Another sad milestone, among many.

CHAPTER 10

"IT'S A PRIVILEGE"

I'll never be able to say with certainty what was going on in her mind, but I can tell you that my own stress kept increasing. My ability to sleep was impacted as I worried about what I was going to do each time she was released – how was I going to keep her safe, manage her dwindling resources, meet her needs, and pleas to "take me home." I wrapped up a business project just at the point that working with her became nearly unmanageable, and we moved our household from Florida to Michigan to be closer to her and better able to deal with all of the churn. She didn't seem to realize the toll that this was taking on me and my husband or other family members. In fact, I learned from another family member that she made up a reason for the move, claiming that our daughter had asked us to come back to Michigan! I never told her anything of the kind. While I'm sure that our daughter is glad to have us in the area, I know that she is also sorry we've left Florida, since she and our granddaughters enjoyed their frequent visits there. No more easy access to the ocean or Disney. Although we were well-organized, especially due to the amazing efforts of my husband, no interstate move is easy, especially in your sixties, and settling in would require months of work.

Adding to the emotional distress I felt was the over-used phrase "it's such a privilege to help someone at this stage of their life." I see this in articles all the time and I've encountered many people who, when I spoke about my mom and our situation, would say things like "it was hard, but I found it such a privilege" to care for their mom/dad in their last days. While probably not intended, it felt like they were saying that they managed a similar situation really well, and even welcomed the opportunity, so there must be something wrong with me. Hearing this made me feel guilty as I struggled with my own frustration with my mom seeming to sit back and let me handle everything from her housing to groceries to making sure bills were paid, and then making snide comments or pouncing on me unkindly when she didn't like something, or worse, literally blaming me for her lack of mobility. Unlike these other folks who spoke of their privilege reverently, my own assessment of the experience included thoughts like "failure and resentment...fear...worry...stress...hard work...just do the right thing no matter what...ensure safety above all else...avoid regrets... high road...do my best."

I resolved to do my best to ensure her safety while also trying to come to terms with the reality that at this stage of her life, nothing was likely to change, and she would never really engage constructively to help with her own life plan. I will say that as this went on and I talked with people more openly about what I was experiencing, I encountered others who talked about the anger and mean behavior of their own parent and how hurtful it was. Just because someone is old, it doesn't necessarily follow that they are sweet and gentle. My instinct is that this phenomenon of anger among the elderly as they face fear and uncertainty is far more common than it may seem, but that it is not written or talked about perhaps out of embarrassment or sadness. Someone I've known for more than twenty years recently told me that her own mother became very nasty to her during her final years and described the time as the worst years of her life. Yet while it was happening, I don't recall her ever mentioning her mom's meanness. Maybe it seemed disloyal and too sad and personal to her, to talk about. And that is so unfortunate, both for the elderly and for their families. I've become convinced that this may be a common occurrence among the aging, for which we might help people become more equipped to handle, if we were more open about it.

To make matters worse, it is also common for people to speak disparagingly about long-term facilities. They're "dumping grounds for old people," "I'd never put my parent in one of those places, they are full of drooling old people," are just a couple of things that I've heard people say. What an unkind way to speak about the elderly and those who care for them. And talk about a guilt inducer! But seriously, what do you do when the parent cannot be alone and needs around the clock care that goes beyond what you can provide? Even if you could devote 100% of your time and resources to this kind of support, it's not always possible for family members to provide the actual care that needs to be given. Some of the maladies that afflict the elderly are extremely debilitating both physically and mentally and difficult to manage and witness. Care facilities don't come with magic wands that can make everything better. It can be devastating to hear people say these things when you're in the midst of trying to do your best to keep your parent safe and well-cared for. I've often wondered if people who make these kinds of comments are really masking their own fear of aging and all that goes with it.

And I take extra, and very personal, exception to these statements. My late sister had been a caring, award-wining nursing home administrator at the time of her death. She was working on a graduate degree in long-term care administration at the School of Aging Studies at the University of South Florida, where I have established an annual scholarship in long-term care administration in her memory. I have been impressed with the faculty and programs at USF, all aimed at better understanding aging and how to support people as they age. Certainly, there is always room for improvement and there are some bad apples. But long-term care is a very real need and carelessly disparaging it and the true heroes who work in these critical roles helps no one.

Families all over the country are flying without a net with elderly loved ones, doing the best they can to navigate through the resource gap and take care of mental and physical health needs. It's exhausting and hard and support from the health care system is limited and complicated to utilize.

Yes, it is unquestionably a privilege and enormous responsibility to help someone navigate their final years, particularly when you are able to connect and reflect and bond, and hopefully ease their passing. But life can be messy and hard and unfair and telling someone who is struggling in the face of this kind of difficulty that this is a privilege is not only simplistic and unhelpful, it is harmful.

Information Central

During my mom's stints in the hospital, rehab, and long-term care, I received frequent texts and phone calls from people asking for updates and saying, "keep me informed." This became another source of stress, particularly during periods in which some new health issue arose. People wanted updates and the need to repeat the story numerous times so that everyone was current added difficulty, especially when accompanied by advice and "did you think of this" kinds of questions.

And of course, the implication behind these questions seemed to be the expectation that I am in 24/7 communication with my mom and support staff. I would get questions from people asking how often I visit my mom or when I last visited her. These questions sometimes made me question myself about whether I was going enough—even though I visited extremely often. And then I realized that some of the people asking such questions visited far less than I did, if at all, and had to remind myself not to read something into the question, and even if criticism was intended, it's not my issue.

When I reported that mom was having a bad day, I'd get "did you ask the doctor about that" or a variety of other questions that seemed to imply to my stressed-out self that I needed to do more or provide even more updates. I urge anyone in a similar situation to do what you can to avoid adding this monkey to your back. Trying to own keeping others informed is too much. Do what you can, but on your own terms and timeframes, and hold people accountable for their own knowledge and for staying connected.

CHAPTER 11

NAVIGATING THE HEALTH CARE SYSTEM: IMPACT OF THE RULES

As the experience with my mom unfolded, I had the opportunity to interact with agencies, companies, health care professionals, and even lawyers as I tried to figure out what to do as the situation evolved. At times it felt like a train wreck in slow motion…a difficult, scary situation and no clear way to make it better.

Rules, rules and more rules

As Mom's situation progressed, I became more aware of different rules and policies related to approved length of hospital stays, and things like the amount of time that must pass before follow-up care can occur in nursing homes. Terms like "left against medical advice (AMA)" carry with them ominous consequences, potentially impacting the patient's physical well-being, possibly the involvement of Adult Protective Services, and maybe even worse, whether a nursing facility will accept a patient who has a history of doing that. As the administrator of the second rehab facility that Mom went to bluntly said to me, " the first rehab facility won't take her back, and if she pulls that here, we won't either, and she will have alienated the two best properties in the area." In other words, if she needs to visit such a facility again in the future, she is seriously limiting her options in a way that could literally impact her living experience, possibly even for the rest of her life. Serious stuff.

While I became aware of all of these rules and policies and guidelines, it would be inaccurate to say that I understand them all or their interdependencies, even after months of engagement. Incredibly, during a period of just over 60 days, Mom's gross expenses passed the $100,000 mark – staggering! And the number grew and grew from there. The prices are incredible. A five-mile ride from the hospital to the rehab center in an ambulance cost $1900!!! When I used a medical transportation company for a similar ride, it was $42. In a period of six months, my mom used the services of two hospitals (four admissions); three nursing home/rehab facilities (four admissions); a transition-to-home service company; a home health care company; an untold number of physical and occupational therapists; and doctors, nurses, and loads of other health care workers with various titles. Oh, and let's not forget the fantastic emergency service personnel! I'm grateful that she had a good Medigap supplement policy and the company she used provides a great website that can be used to monitor claims and Explanation of Benefits documents. Without that, I truly don't know where we'd be. As it was, watching funds disappear without really having clarity on what was ahead made was extremely nerve-wracking. I was determined that this situation would not harm our own financial viability, but there were a lot of unknowns.

Adult Protective Services

Upon learning that my mother had left the rehab center and returned to the home we own, we called Adult Protective Services. She had disowned her family and we did not believe she was acting in her own best interests. While people tend to think of APS as the place to call when concerned about an adult being harmed at the hands of another person, they are also a resource when you fear that someone may be neglecting themselves in some way or creating a harmful environment for themselves. When we first called, we didn't know that she had skipped taking appropriate discharge steps, but we were concerned that it was unlikely that she had made arrangements for even simple things like groceries, since she wasn't speaking to anyone in the family, and would not answer the phone.

In hindsight, all of our concerns proved to be true (and then some) and we appreciated the care that the APS case worker took in gathering and documenting the information. We were told that they would look into it further and that they would get back to us within the next couple of weeks. We learned later that day that they had immediately engaged with the first rehab center, at which point the full details about the Thelma and Louise break-out also came to light for all of us.

Unbelievably, we found ourselves calling them again the next day to alert them to the fact that Mom had been transported to the hospital within 18 hours of leaving the rehab center against medical advice, and with zero discharge planning. We again were grateful for the thoughtful, understanding person with whom we spoke. It was surreal that we were in this situation, and we felt it important to document things both for Mom's protection and our own.

A few days later, we were contacted by a caseworker at the hospital, who seemed to be trying to get to the bottom of what was going on with Mom. I don't really know what Mom told her but went through the entire mess with her over the phone. She told me that she would have to file her own report with APS, which I wholeheartedly supported.

Perhaps because she left the hospital for another rehab center, rather than going home alone, and there was a plan for her safety, we did not hear anything further from APS, and as of this writing, we have not contacted them again ourselves, but we remain grateful for their support.

Programs to help people stay home

I was interested to learn about a couple of programs that are available to those with limited income to use for some financial support while in assisted living or in services to help stay in the home. There are limits, of course, and waiting lists but I looked into applying when I hoped I could convince my mom to try assisted living. I learned that you need to be no more than 60 days away from having less than $2000 in assets to start the application process and that would have been the case if Mom moved to assisted living. Since she would not pursue that option, it would take a few more months before we could apply, since her three-day-per-week home care was not as expensive as 24/7 assisted living or around-the-clock home care.

We planned to apply again when her funds were spent down to the designated point and hoped that she would eventually qualify for this support. Taking this kind of additional financial hit for a sustained period would be a huge concern to my husband and me this early in our own retirement.

Finally, we were unable to get a clear answer about the role of credit card debt in the determination of assets. Should we pay off her debt, she would reach the remaining assets number immediately, but the agency also speaks about a "look-back" period in which large payments are reviewed as part of the determination process. No one seemed able to tell me if paying off her debt would harm her application, so we did not do it. Of course, what that meant is that a situation was created in which fully paying off this debt with her own resources ultimately became completely impossible. This was troubling, and more so, given her propensity to charge things. She would soon have no assets and growing debt. We did keep making monthly payments, of course, until the day came at which we needed to contact the company in an effort to work things out.

Another problem with these programs is that you cannot apply for them until you are almost out of money, which can result in a further erosion of health and capabilities that might have been staved off by earlier access to more help. A Catch 22 for sure. Having more assistance has the potential to bolster one's strength and safety in the home. By delaying that or cutting back on the assistance one really needs in order to manage finances, the result may actually result in diminishing chances of staying in the home safely longer term.

Because we hadn't quite reached the targeted asset level, we never got the chance to complete our applications for these programs to help her at home and instead it was necessary to apply for Medicaid when her mobility became so compromised that it was finally clear to all, with the possible exception of Mom, that returning home was not remotely viable and she needed to move into long-term care. And that was the point when we reached another sad milestone. We needed to seriously make plans to sell the house to which she longed to return.

Legal implications

One of the most difficult aspects of this journey has been my mom's treatment of me and my siblings. Her decision to toss us aside and stated intent to make ill-conceived plans to move into an apartment or hotel and ultimately leave the first rehab facility against medical advice was heartbreaking. Whether in "right mind" or not, these actions required steps that I never envisioned taking with my mom.

Because she lived in a house owned by my husband and me, told us she was going to leave, then reversed that by ultimately moving back in without telling us and concurrently misleading the rehab facility, while also failing to ensure a plan to keep safe, we were very worried about her safety, as well as the possibility of liability for ourselves. In addition to making a report with Adult Protective Services, we had no choice but to consult an elder care attorney.

We'd had a couple of people suggest that becoming her guardian might be necessary. While I have power of attorney, I've come to realize that this really doesn't help much when a parent is in situations like ours, in which the parent is coherent (or at least seems to be) and generally able to articulate opinions, even while making decisions that those close to them can see are not in their best interests or may not even be fact-based. And when the parent gives people erroneous information about their support network and finances, it becomes even harder for others to see the issues that family members can see. All this said, I was very reluctant to pursue guardianship. Such a course of action would undoubtedly make my mother very angry and inevitably make communication even more challenging. And discussing this with an attorney underscored that this can be a slow process. I just didn't want to do this.

However, the situation with the house was particularly concerning. We were advised that we needed documentation should we need to evict my mom. Evict my mom!!! What a horrific thought and something I would never have imagined in a million years would be on the table. But our concern about having Mom living in the house and refusing to have any help was dangerous to her, as well as created risks to the house itself. If we could not find a way to address some of these issues, eviction could indeed be needed, which would then put a bigger spotlight on the guardianship question. What a nightmare! With assistance from an attorney, we did send her a letter documenting her own stated intentions to move out, along with our sadness to be in this pickle and attempting to outline some of the ramifications that could occur if we didn't work this out. While we also tried to make it clear our primary interest was in working things out, she claimed that we were doing this because we wanted her out of the house. And Louise was right there, reinforcing these conclusions. How did something that we did with the very best of intentions and intended to help her, end up being turned against us in this ugly way? All we had ever wanted was for her to be safe and minimize her worries.

As time went on, this issue dissipated somewhat. I think the turning point may have been the scary night that she directly experienced that even together, my brother and I could not really help her get up and down in her house, and she had to be hospitalized. We clearly tried and she saw that with her own eyes. While she didn't stop saying that she wanted to go home, she also began to acknowledge a little more often that she just didn't have enough help to be there on her own.

I've read that life comes in chapters, and it will always sadden me that my mom's final chapter included so much pain and unhappiness, both for her, and for her family. Some of it was needless, some of it was unavoidable, and all of it was more difficult given the complexities of the health care facilities, programs, and systems and the associated extreme financial implications that constantly needed navigating. And the paperwork was incredible, as literally hundreds of forms, explanations of benefits, and documents required for each medical facility needed to be perused, filled out, or filed. Thank goodness so much is electronic or online now.

I'm keenly aware that, despite these challenges, we're among the lucky ones, and I'm grateful for that. And despite all of the challenges, I'm especially grateful for my mom and my dad, their lives and all the experiences we shared during nearly seven decades.

EPILOGUE

As I said at the outset, I know that my parents would probably be unhappy with me for sharing what I am sure they would consider our family's "dirty laundry." And so much of this describes experiences that most, including me, would rightly describe as private and intimate. But it's all real life. The reality is that aging can be brutal and hard, and I worry that by masking descriptions of the difficulty of this experience with euphemisms like "it's a privilege," we make it harder collectively to understand that the current state of services is inadequate and just doesn't cut it. Furthermore, we risk underutilization of services that **do** exist when we suggest that people "should" take of the elderly themselves, as if there is something shameful about using nursing facilities.

My mother's treatment of me and my brothers was, at times, breathtakingly heartbreaking, second only in sadness, to the death of my younger sister when she was only 37. It's easy to understand why losing autonomy and needing to rely on others for even simple things would make a person mad. It's hard, though, to be on the receiving end of that anger, even when you know it's displaced. There remains a part of me that will always hope that she didn't really mean all the unfortunate things she said and did in the twilight of her life.

I'm going to cling to that hope as I celebrate and remember the many very special things about my mom, especially her amazing artistic talent. As I end this story, it seems fitting to recount some of the things that made her unique and for which I am grateful to have lasting, positive memories.

My parents worked together on several small businesses during their life together, including a heating oil distribution business, an A&W drive-in, a convenience store, and one that bore her name, Arlene's Pop Shoppe. She worked in these businesses and helped in lots of ways, keeping records, answering phones, even flipping burgers; but in each case, her special contribution was in using her immense artistic talent to design and paint signage.

That talent also manifested itself over the years in beautiful oil paintings portraying many subjects, including a very special painting of herself and her sister, hand-in-hand with their grandfather. She made incredible hooked rugs and wall hangings, and created amazing, detailed quilts, even one that commemorated the September 11 attacks on the United States. She had fun calling herself a "hooker" in reference to her rug-hooking years and once even demonstrated her craft in costume at Greenfield Village, part of The Henry Ford, in Dearborn, Michigan.

She was an accomplished knitter and seamstress and used those skills to create sweaters, clothes, and blankets for her family. She managed to perfectly replicate an outfit I was drooling over in Seventeen magazine when I was a teenager. Wandering through fabric stores looking at patterns, material, and buttons was one of her favorite things to do. I liked doing these things with her when I was a kid, although I didn't have even a fraction of her talent.

Her artistic DNA can be found in several of her grandchildren and great-grandchildren, and we are all grateful that her creativity will continue through them.

Mom loved dogs, especially dachshunds, and had several, including Pretzel, Domino, and Speckles. She kept an eye on pet adoption sites, especially to check out the dachshunds. She collected dolls and was an avid reader, with her Kindle always close-at-hand. She enjoyed cooking shows and detective stories (especially those starring Tom Selleck!) and shopping for new gadgets on Amazon.

Her challenges in her later years do not define her but do illustrate the difficulties families have in supporting loved ones as they age. It is in the spirit of perhaps providing some insight that may be useful to other families that I share this story.

Ultimately, I could not fulfill her request to take her home. I did my best to take care of her and to keep her safe as long as possible. As I made her final arrangements, I was sad for many reasons, but also because she and my dad would not be together. Dad had made a special request for disposition of his ashes that was different from what my mom had requested. They were ok with this, as they each had their own reasons, but it bothered me that they wouldn't be together. And my sister was buried in Florida, more than a thousand miles away. So, when I arrived at the cemetery and entered the mausoleum where mom would be, I was astonished and pleased to see that mom's mother's (my grandmother) best friend and her husband are in the same mausoleum, literally right across the hall! So, while she hadn't gone back to her house, she has friends in the neighborhood.

Rest well, Mom.